131
Dirty Talk Examples

Learn How To Talk Dirty with These
Simple Phrases That Drive Your Lover
Wild & Beg You For Sex Tonight

Elizabeth Cramer
Copyright© 2013 by Elizabeth Cramer

Publisher: Living Plus Healthy Publishing

ISBN-13: 978-1494355005

ISBN-10: 1494355000

Disclaimer

The Publisher has strived to be as accurate and complete as possible in the creation of this book. While all attempts have been made to verify information provided in this publication, the Publisher assumes no responsibility for errors, omissions, or contrary interpretation of the subject matter herein. Any perceived slights of specific persons, peoples, or organizations are unintentional.

This book is not intended for use as a source of legal, business, accounting or financial advice. All readers are advised to seek services of competent professionals in the legal, business, accounting, and finance fields.

The information in this book is not intended or implied to be a substitute for professional medical advice, diagnosis or treatment. All content contained in this book is for general information purposes only. Always consult your healthcare provider before carrying on any health program.

Table of Contents

Introduction

The concept of dirty talk can elicit a variety of different reactions in a person, sometimes all at once. Some people think of the concept of dirty talk and giggle internally (or externally), others get embarrassed and start acting nervously like the person sitting across the way can tell exactly what they are thinking about, while still others get the anticipatory tightening of things low in the body, knowing that the juicy bits are about to come (pun intended).

Many people think about talking dirty, but few people ever talk about it. It's a deliciously taboo topic, even in today's free information society; while you can read about a friend's every second of every day on Facebook, sex is a topic that few are comfortable discussing openly and in public; sure a person may tell their close friend about their latest escapades, but few will bring it up as part of a normal out in public conversation, unless euphemisms are used. Sex happens. Every minute of every day, someone somewhere is having sex, and many of those people are talking dirty to each other while they're doing it.

There are others, though, who may want to spice up their love life with the addition of dirty talk, longing to hear certain words or phrases whispered, moaned, growled, or simply uttered but they just plain don't know how to get started. They may even be a little embarrassed to bring it up, because they fear how their partner will take it, thinking that "oh, so and so doesn't think our sex life is good enough" or worried about whether or not their partner will take them seriously or some other such nonsense.

But what we call dirty talk is just plain erotic, and there's no shame in wanting to hear softly moaned words, begging, pleading, or demanding. There's the thrill that comes from the taboo, saying the words out loud, and there's the difference that comes from hearing your partner tell you want they want to do to you, and what you want them to do which can also work to ensure a more satisfying sex life, as it provides your partner with a look into your head, so that you can both get exactly what you want, when you want it.

How many times have you had a partner that did something that really detracted from your experience, like wearing nothing but their socks? Instead of telling them, loose them or this isn't happening, this too can be turned around, with something as simple as "lose all the clothes; I want to see you completely naked." By saying exactly what you want, when you want it, you are able to enhance the experience for not only you, but your partner as well.

Men and women want to know that they are desired, and they both have their insecurities, whether they are worried that something is jiggling that shouldn't be, or something isn't jiggling that should. Every single person in the world has their own hang-ups, and with the proper wording, anyone can be assured that not only are they wonderful, and sexy, but that they are desirable for who they are as well.

The other thing to consider is that you are doing one of the most intimate things you can with another human being, and if you can't talk to them about what you want, you aren't as close as you would like to be, or as you could be.

Why Dirty Talk Is Erotic

There are a few different reasons why dirty talk is erotic, and it's not just because of the taboo surrounding it. Men like descriptions to go along with their visuals, and women like to imagine and fantasize; it's just the way that the sexes are wired. There's nothing strange, abnormal, or weird about it. Everyone has "dirty" thoughts, and like Mel Gibson's character found out in "What Women Want" there's a lot more going through our brains during sex that isn't verbalized.

The first thing to understand is that dirty talk isn't dirty. There's nothing shameful or wrong about it, and once that's understood, it doesn't take away the feeling of taboo, due to the society that we live in today, but rather serves to enhance it; there's a feeling of "I'm saying these things out loud, and it's okay," but there's also the feeling of "I'm so glad that (insert name of person here) can't hear me now; they wouldn't believe that these words are coming out of my mouth." If you don't like the phrasing "dirty talk" there are many different ways of phrasing it, like naughty talk for example.

Men and women are hard-wired differently. Men like to hear, while women like to visualize, and that's completely natural too. A man wants to hear what their partner wants done to them, or wants to do for them before it's done. Hearing the words, screamed, moaned, whimpered, or whispered just flat out does it for most men. Women like to hear the words and imagine what those words or phrases will mean to them, how their partner will react, or how something will feel, even seconds or milliseconds beforehand, giving their brains time to process the possibilities, thus heightening the sensations.

In addition, it provides an additional feeling of closeness between the two parties, because you are not only sharing your bodies with each other at that point, but you are also sharing your thoughts, providing an even further melding than would otherwise occur.

Talking dirty isn't just about saying what one person wants to do to, or for, the other, but it's also about encouragement, and about polite, yet sexy, redirection. One example of redirection was provided earlier, taking what could be an awkward and slightly emasculating statement and turning it into something that really serves to stroke the…ego of the other person. It works to make the other person feel more secure, and as a result, more confident, and more sexy, which in turn assures that the person is less stuck inside their own head and more right there experiencing what is going on, instead of worrying, fretting, or simply not being as into it as they could be.

Sex is wonderful, amazing, incredible, and mind blowing, and there is no reason that two people should not be able to talk openly and freely, if only between themselves, if nowhere else, about exactly what they want, how they want it, when they want it, while still feeling sexy, confident, and above all, desired by their partner.

How To Get Started

The first step in changing your ways, regardless of whether it is rearranging the furniture, talking to your boss about that promotion, or talking dirty to your partner is always the hardest. In order to make a change, a person must have several things, the desire to affect change, the drive to make it happen, and the follow through to do so, regardless of the change that is being made.

If you're not comfortable simply diving right in and trying a phrase or two, that's okay. It's natural to be a little shy, when although our society uses sex as a selling tool, it's implied, rather than overtly stated. In some topics, it is far easier to imply than to have to state something, and this is one of those topics. Diving right in is not for everyone, but there are definitely ways to ease in slowly, going a little deeper, and pushing a little further each time.

One way to lead into talking dirty in the bedroom is to start out by bringing up the subject outside of the bedroom. While there are some places that will not be the appropriate setting for this conversation, there are many others that can present themselves. If you don't just want to come out and ask them what their feelings on the subject are, bring it up as though you heard about something your buddy did with their partner, or say that you were reading an article on the topic, or even reading a novel that mentioned it, and ask what they think of that. In this manner, the attention is redirected from the fact that you are asking about how they feel about dirty talk, but to the idea of dirty talk in a particular context, and that depersonalization can give a person the jump they need to get started.

Another method is to try one or two phrases out on your partner mid coitus and see how they react. If there is a noticeably favorable response, you can work up from there, working a greater volume in each time. If that's still too bold straight out, that's fine, a different method is to start working it in to your daily life through other communication mediums. Many of the different phrases provided at the end of this article can be used as "one-offs," possible things to say that are quite normal, but don't have to lead into more talking. This method often leads to further talking and discussion, however, both from the initial thrill that is experienced from finally saying something like this out loud, but also from the subsequent thrill of seeing how your partner reacts, and a desire to see them react that way again.

An email sent after a night of carnal pleasure is one way to test the waters; start out by telling your partner how much you enjoyed when they did x, y, or z, and be descriptive. We're not in kindergarten anymore; saying "I enjoyed when you put your thing in my thing" just will not cut it, and will serve as even more of a potential embarrassment than anything else. Use the names of your body parts, and theirs, that you learned in school, or use slang terms or colorful colloquialisms, but do not be vague. See how they respond, and go from there; while there is a very small possibility that they will not be receptive to receiving this type of email, the likelihood of receiving a response in kind is high. This can be done via text or serve as a starting point for phone sex as well.

Dirty talk done through the medium of text is referred to as sexting, and may provide the easiest way to get started, along with email, as it allows the initiator to do so from in front of a screen, behind a keyboard, offering the illusion of anonymity, in spite of the fact that you already know the person you are writing to.

Phone sex is another way to start, discussing sexual or sensual activities over the phone with your partner. This is best done in a private, quiet place, one where you feel perfectly comfortable, with not only your surroundings, but with anyone who may be in the vicinity. For example, someone might be comfortable initiating this while knowing their best friend is in the next room over, but they may not feel comfortable with their relatives in the next room. Comfort level is key, and as long as you are comfortable, the acts, the words, and the written text will become more and more comfortable as time goes by.

Oftentimes, all that a person is waiting for is for the other person to say something first, and the more frequently you do so, the more like a second nature it will become, and the more comfortable you will be with it. Dirty talk adds spice, variety, and can be highly erotic, but perhaps more importantly, it should be enjoyable. The goal is not to add something that makes you uncomfortable, but to add something that both you and your partner can thoroughly enjoy.

What To Say – 131 Erotic Things to Say to Your Partner

There are all different kinds of things that you can say to your partner, some more tame than others, referred to as softcore and hardcore dirty talk. Softcore dirty talk is less vulgar, and more general, while hardcore is more explicit. The following are 131 different things that can be said to your partner before, during, or after sex. They are not in any particular order. Of course, when to say the phrase depends on how the phrase should be said, and it is important to tailor the phrase to the situation at hand (like using past tense after the fact, future tense before, and present tense during; remember, bad grammar can turn a sexy phrase into something awkward, and this whole thing is about avoiding any awkwardness while still having a very good time).

The type of dirty talk you use with your sweetie will depend on the person, what they like, and how comfortable you are uttering certain words or phrases, though simply talking isn't the whole shebang, moans, coos, whimpers, and gasps play a part as well. The point is to show them that you are into them, with every word, utterance, sound, and movement. (If you're not 100% into it, chances are that you shouldn't be there in the first place.) If you are too nervous about saying something out loud straight away, practice saying it to yourself when no one else is around until you are no longer made uncomfortable by it, or unsure of doing so.

Getting In The Mood

1. I want you.

Plain, simple, and sweet, this serves to show your partner that you want them, no one else, and it's all you can think of currently. Not only is this a real ego booster, but it's a simple and honest statement of desire, and it is that honest, raw statement that makes it really do the trick.

2. Damn, I've missed you.

This shows your partner how much you care, no matter how long it's been since you were last together. The soft emphasis of the curse word at the beginning helps to drive the point home. It shows that you have missed their touch, their presence, their smile, the way they move, how they feel, everything about them, and how much you want them still. It's an incredibly erotic statement to make, no matter how long you may have been together.

3. You're the sexiest thing I have ever seen.

With statements like this, you serve to confirm that your partner is the only one on your mind at the time, and that you desire them for who they are, and more than that, you genuinely appreciate everything they have to offer. You show your partner that it is them, and only them, that you want, and that they are the most desirable person you can think of at this time.

4. You smell so good.

5. Your hair smells so good.

6. Your scent is amazing.

With this comment you are allying any potential fears, worries, or concerns that they may have that may be preventing them from being fully in the moment, thereby ensuring that they are right there with you, intensifying their pleasure, and as a result, enhancing yours. By making statements like this, you ensure that you are both paying attention to nothing but each other, that there is nothing else on either of your minds, which in turn heightens awareness of the situation you are in, which turns into increased arousal.

7. You amaze me.

This is another form of validation, showing in words just a small amount of how spectacular you think they are. You want to be sure that your partner knows in each and every possible way how much you desire them, and how truly special you think they are. So many people forget this aspect; just because they should know that they are special to you, does not mean in any way, shape, or form, that you should not tell them every chance you get.

8. I wish I could hold you all day long.

Simple, sweet, and succinct, it expresses a desire of more time spent together, wrapped up in each other, basking in each other's arms.

9. I love it when you pull my hair.

Again, by calling specific attention to an action that you really enjoy, you guarantee that action for a repeat performance, giving them confidence that they are doing something right, and ensuring that you get that same feeling again. This action can be hair pulling, or it can be something else, any action at all. The point is to draw their attention to that specific action, and show how much you love it, guaranteeing that the particular action will come up more and more frequently.

10. You are so pretty.

11. You are so hot.

12. Your skin feels so soft.

13. You look so sexy in that underwear.

14. Your eyes are so beautiful.

15. Your lips taste like honey.

16. I want to feel your nails in my skin.

Telling someone what you want, what will heighten your pleasure serves to provide a pleasure boost in and of itself, and it provides them with helpful direction, as opposed to them attempting to read your mind as to what you actually want. Some people like a little pain with their pleasure, and getting the right balance, when coupled with the right wording, serves to enhance not only the physical sensations, but the mental sensations associated with the action as well.

17. It drives me crazy when you look at me that way.

Again, in this manner you are showing that it is them and only them that is turning you on. You want that person, and when they give you that look, whatever that look is, it just makes you want them more. You want them, and only them, and they don't have to worry that the look they are giving you makes their face look weird, is just plain awkward, or anything of that nature. It takes away that niggling doubt and worry in the back of their mind, serving to keep them more fully into the situation itself.

18. The feeling of you overpowering me, dominating me, is like nothing else.

This is for those particular partners who are on the submissive side, if only in bed, and who really appreciate being topped by the right person. It doesn't have to be an intense or a rough overpowering, just showing your partner that you really like it when they are in charge of what happens next.

19. Tell me your fantasies, down to every detail.

There is something incredibly personal about speaking your fantasies out loud, and more so that you are telling them to another person, a person that you already have an intense physical connection with. This sharing is hot in and of itself, and further enhanced by the particular conversation topic; the more detail provided, the better it can be.

20. Shut up and kiss me.

This shows that the time for talking about the mundane, the everyday, and the ordinary is done, and there should be one thing, and one thing only, on your partner's mind, and that is getting lost in you. It may also be used to quite literally get your partner to shut up, or to distract them from doing something that you aren't really enjoying and providing a nice, smooth transition into something else.

21. I want you to undress and wait for me in the bedroom.

By providing these two commands in conjunction with the other, this can lead to one of a few things. It serves to take away control of the partner, even temporarily, and it allows you to leave them there, waiting, wondering when you will be there, wondering what will happen tonight, and causing the imagination to go in all different directions, increasing the anticipation of both parties.

22. It's my turn to make the rules tonight.

By making this declarative statement, you are showing that you are taking control for the night, offering a further sense of eagerness, tinged with desire, and mixed with a tad bit of apprehension, as they will not know what you have in mind for the evening, but they will have already started to think about the different possible things that could be coming their way.

During Foreplay

23. You look so sexy when you do that.

This is really good for those particularly self-conscious moments, showing that in spite of how paranoid your partner may be about a particular act, pose, or look, that you still find them to be desirable, regardless of whatever hang-ups they may have. This is especially true of those couples who have been together for longer periods of time, as due to that duration, they may no longer feel as desirable as they did when the two of you first got together, and while you may still desire them just as much as you did the first day, the validation provided by hearing those words out loud is always a good boost.

24. I want to feel you in my mouth.

Telling someone exactly what you want heightens the pleasure gained from the particular action, and shows that you are just as into it as they are. It also provides a stunning visual of what will come next, ensuring that the mental imagery is just as strong as the physical sensation and that each one funnels into the other, serving to enhance both.

25. You taste so good.

This is another good one for those self-conscious moments, easing any concerns that your partner may have about whether or not you are doing something because you want to do it, or if you are doing so just because they want you to. It shows that you're right there with them, and loving every minute of it. It's surprising how much of a difference this one simple phrase can make to both peace of mind and increased enjoyment. It serves to get the other person out of their head completely and right back into the current action going on.

26. Your pussy tastes so good.

27. Your juices taste so good.

28. I love the things you do with your tongue.

This serves as another way to point your partner in the right direction, showing them what you like, or what you prefer, with your vocalizations, ensuring that those are the things that they keep in mind for the next time, and providing a polite way to take the things you don't like out of rotation. In place of talking about the different ways that they use their tongue that you especially enjoy, you can substitute fingers, legs, arms, lips, teeth, and so on.

29. I want you so bad.

By flat out telling someone you want them, you are not only stroking their ego, showing them that they are desirable as a human being, but also that it isn't some fantasy going through your head. You want them and not some other random person. It's a heady feeling to know that you are desired above all else, and that feeling will translate into other aspects of the particular experience that you are currently engaging in with your partner.

30. Your wish is my command.

This serves as another way to give up control and give it to your partner, if only in the bedroom, and if only for this night. In doing so, you are showing that you trust that they will not ask anything unreasonable, irrational, or potentially harmful of them. The idea that someone will do anything for you, if you will only utter it is a heady feeling indeed and it serves to increase the anticipation behind any thought, action, or deed taken from that point on.

31. Play with yourself for me. I want to watch.

This will appeal to the person with the voyeuristic side, the person for whom being watched is a complete turn on, and even if the person does not believe they are voyeuristic, they will find themselves getting turned on just seeing the other person getting turned on as they watch.

32. Do you like it when I touch myself here?

This makes item number 31 a bit more interactive, asking what aspects best appeal to your partner, and giving more information not only on how they get themselves off (providing pointers), but also letting you know what they like best.

33. Kiss me there. (With each there point to a spot).

By turning this into an order, the power rush when your partner moves to obey your every whim, showing that you are in control adds a further sense of anticipation to their each and every move.

34. Lick every inch of me.

Another order, showing again that, for right now at least, you are in control, and offering an increased sense of anticipation for you, imagining exactly how they will do so, where they will start, and attempting to guess what will come next.

35. I could spend hours between your legs; teasing you, sucking you, tasting you.

The visuals that this evokes, the imagery, is enough to tighten things low in your partner's body, making the sensations once you go back to your task that much more intense, because they are imagining this going on for far longer than it is.

36. Tell me how you touch yourself.

This is another variant on number 31, using the descriptive imagery to paint a picture and serving to increase the sense of urgency for things to escalate from where they currently are. It can also serve to show you which words or phrases that your partner may like; by making note of the words they use, you are able to see which words they prefer, and can consequently turn around and use those same words back on them, offering an additional boost.

37. Grab my head and force me closer.

By telling your partner what you want them to do, you are showing again that you are giving control to them, and that you trust them to not use that power to cause any adverse harm, or to cause any issues with your body, and saying that you believe they know your body's limitations.

38. Your body is mine tonight.

This is a possessive declaration; showing that you belong to your partner, and they will do whatever they want, manipulate your body however they want, and give or suspend pleasure at any time, simply for the enjoyment and anticipation of both parties.

39. You have no idea what I am going to do to you tonight.

40. I always get what I want, and what I want right now is you.

This statement is not only full of confidence, but by showing confidence in yourself, you are also showing confidence in your partner and the certainty that they want you just as much as you want them, and because of that, will give up their control and play the subservient, at least this once.

41. You are so wet.

42. I adore how naughty you are.

This works to validate your partner as well, showing them that you like what they are doing, and how they are doing it, and that you want them to continue. It takes away the second guessing, so you don't leave your partner trying something new and then fretting about whether or not it was enjoyed, or appreciated.

43. Your tits feel so good.

44. My cock feels so good between your tits.

45. You will do what I say tonight.

This is almost a continuation of number forty, as it allows for not only a punishment aspect if something is disobeyed, but also offers a potential power shift, which spices things up in and of itself, by changing the game around a bit. Statements like this work best when used with a tone that will brook no argument, showing clearly exactly who has decided to take charge at this time.

46. I'm your slave for the night. Tell me what you want me to do for you.

For many, this conjures up images of a partner in a slave's costume, forced to do anything asked of them, and with that imagery comes increased titillation. It is the ultimate concept of giving up complete and total control.

47. Look down. Tell me what you see; describe it to me.

By having your partner watch what is happening, and then describe it, the auditory and visual stimulation that will result, when combined with the physical sensations already being felt, serve to expand the experience for both parties. This audio track serves to enhance the pleasure of both parties, and may also be used as a way to offer a shift in roles, with the partner who is describing things changes from describing what is occurring to what they want to happen next.

48. Not yet; you haven't teased me enough yet. Make me beg.

This shows that you are asking to be submissive for the duration of the encounter, putting your partner in sole control; it is completely up to them how much, and how long, the teasing will be, and whether or not they give you what you beg for is completely up to you.

49. You can have any hole you want.

A phrase of this nature shows that there is an explicit level of trust in the relationship, and that there is no doubt in your mind that not only will they not cause you harm, but also that they will make the experience a particularly enjoyable one for you.

50. Suck on my balls.

This command to a partner shows a high level of trust with this especially sensitive and easily damaged area of the body; it tells their partner how deep the confidence that no harm will befall them is, while ensuring that they are the recipient of what is described as a most pleasant feeling.

51. I am so hard for you.

52. You make me so hard.

53. Look at how ready I am.

This triggers the visual aspect, inviting your partner to look, really look, and not just see, how much you desire them; a powerful aphrodisiac. By drawing attention to the evidence of your desire, you are ensuring your partner is right there in the moment with you. They are fully aware of what their actions are doing to you, and they are able to see how truly desired they really are.

54. Feel how ready I am for you.

This is a slight variation on number three, moving it from the visual to the physical, making it interactive, and combining the words with the visual allows for that extra shiver of anticipation. It is one thing to see how much a person physically affects another person, however to touch that physical manifestation of their desire for you takes it up to a whole different level of anticipation.

55. You want me to fuck you, don't you?

56. Do you want to feel my cock in your pussy?

57. I can't wait to feel you inside of me.

This further proves that you want your partner, and you want them right now; this serves to show the eagerness you feel, and prove that you are in the moment with your partner themselves.

During Intercourse

58. I'm going to do you right now; do you want it in your pussy or your ass?

This type of declarative statement clearly defines which person is the dominant in that particular situation, though by allowing the partner to pick the orifice that will be used, shows that the partner still has a certain amount of free will during the course of the actions to come. The partner may never know what the dominant will give them a choice in next, allowing the different possibilities to spread through their mind, enhancing the experience.

59. I want to fuck you.

This is similar to one of our earlier statements, however, this shows that you are taking charge of the situation; you are the dominant, and it has all of the implications that are associated with this particular concept.

60. Remember how you made me scream last week? Do it again.

This, our last and final phrasing for this report, shows your partner that you really enjoyed last week, which you've been thinking about it since then, and you really want a repeat performance of the act with them and them alone. The idea that you have been (continuously) thinking about that particular act all week, or whatever variation of time (day, etc.) you add into this particular phrasing, shows not only how much you genuinely enjoyed it, but also that you haven't been able to get them off your mind.

61. That feels incredible; please don't stop.

Though it may seem like a tame phrase, it does several things. First, it provides validation that your partner is doing something so very, very right, and second, by saying please, it puts them in control of the situation. In addition, by putting them in control, you are showing them that you trust them enough to give up that control. Six simple words, yet so very sexy.

62. This feels so good, doesn't it?

63. Just like that.

With these three little words, you are showing that you like what is being done to you, and in doing so, are providing them with incentive to keep going. Encouragement for doing something right is never a bad thing, especially while having sex with your partner. You want to ensure that all those things that you love are going to continue to occur, and that your partner is not in any way confused about what it is that you are really enjoying as a result of their specific actions.

64. Don't stop.

Pretty much exactly what it sounds like. You're telling them that they're doing something right, and that they should continue. This also serves to bring specific attention to a particular action that you especially enjoy, ensuring that it will happen again in the future. Remember, it's always those absolutely electric and intense feelings of pleasure that you want to continue, and your partner cannot read your mind; it is important to show them through words, moans, sighs, and body language how very right a particular thing is that they are doing.

65. Harder!

Many guys, whether subconsciously or not, will treat a girl like she's going to break, and this shows that you're really into it, that you won't break, and that you can take whatever they can dish out. This breaks down that particular mindset, whether or not they realize that it is present, and as such, the more primitive and animalistic sides will come out in both of you, turning something familiar into something far more primal.

66. Turn over.

While these two simple words may not seem like much, they conjure up a myriad of images as to what could occur very soon, heightening the anticipation of what may come. The longer between the words being uttered, the action being performed and the next action being taken, the more likely the level of arousal will rise in great proportion.

67. It turns me on so much when you pin me down.

People want to know that they are desired; by telling them a specific action that makes you desire them more, you are not only providing a confidence boost, but also showing them that you don't want the relationship to end. By using this particular type of phrasing, you are also serving to tie the action to that specific person; it is when they specifically do something, it causes a different reaction in you.

68. You love it when I am inside you, don't you?

69. I love the feeling you inside of me.

This shows your partner that you are not faking it; you want them, you love how they feel, you can't imagine anything better than that at that moment. It is everything that you want. You cannot think of anything that you enjoy the feel of more at that particular moment in time.

70. I don't think there is anything hotter than watching your face when you come.

This shows that giving your partner pleasure gives you great pleasure in return; with it also comes a sense of accomplishment, and satisfaction at a job well done. It also serves to provide encouragement that they are not making a face that looks like a deranged squirrel, but that they still look like someone attractive and desirable, regardless of the face they themselves are making at that particular point and time.

71. Doggie style feels incredible with you.

Any position can be inserted at the beginning of this particular phrase, accomplishing several things; first, you are stroking the ego by mentioning them specifically, and second, you are telling them what position you really liked out of however many you may have happened to go through that round. The more elaboration gone into in regards to the position you have chosen to discuss, the better, as it serves to provide the verbal confirmation of the physical sensations that you are both experiencing, and the more descriptive you get, the greater the enhancement possible.

72. There is something so insanely hot about pinning you down.

This shows your partner that the very act of performing certain acts on them, to them, or for them, is an incredibly erotic experience for you, further validating that you want to be there with them in that moment.

73. No one has ever made me come as hard as you do.

While yes, this is a comparative statement, and you will typically want to stay away from these, as many comparative statements will not come out the way they are intended, this serves to inflate your partner's ego quite a bit by telling them that they are the best you have had, which in turn implies that you want to continue getting exactly what they have to give to you.

74. You like it when I spread my legs for you and take you in, don't you?

By speaking of the actions that are occurring you are providing an audio track for the visuals that are going on in front of your partner's face, increasing their desire twofold. This isn't to say that a running monologue should be going the entire time (unless you and your partner are into that thing – here's where "Shut up and kiss me can come in handy too, if the length of time a description goes on provides too much of a distraction), but to bring in a few descriptive phrases of exactly what is going on at the current time will serve to heighten the experience.

75. Maybe you should spank me; I've been very, very naughty.

This not only tells your partner what you want, but phrases it in such away as though it appears that they have made the decision on their own, but due to the phrasing, the desire to do so was subconsciously placed in their brain. They are more likely to take it and run with it at this point, and you are more likely to get exactly what you are craving.

76. I want to suck your cock until you come.

Short and sweet, and perfect if you love giving head. It's never turned down, and to show the initiative and the desire to do so of your own volition really enhances the act itself. While there are some people who love performing this act, many of those people tend not to say anything because the equivalent is not often reciprocated; if you enjoy it, do it, regardless of whether or not there is any form of "tit for tat." Remember, you are there because you enjoy experiencing your partner; there's no attempting to trade one thing for another. Get enjoyment out of the fact that you are doing something you enjoy, and enjoyment from the fact that your partner is really enjoying themselves and go from there.

77. Get on top.

Similar to telling your partner to turn over, telling them to get on top provides a wide variety of different images, and different possible ways to do so; with both partners imagining the different ways this could happen, it really boosts the sensations.

78. I want you to ride me hard.

The power of telling your partner what you want to happen next, what you want to do next, or what you want them to do next, acts as a powerful aphrodisiac, showing them that you desire them, which in turn increases your desire as you see their desire increase.

79. You are my naughty little girl.

80. You are my naughty little slut.

81. Are you my naughty little bitch?

This will depend on if your partner is okay with being called a bitch, but when used in this manner, it becomes a term of endearment, and if the answer given is yes, additional pleasure can then be given to them as a reward for being "good." It is important to note that regardless of whether you use the term bitch or a different term, the naughty words that are used as terms of endearment in the bedroom should stay in the bedroom.

82. You love it when I fuck you hard, don't you?

83. I love fucking you.

There is no simpler way to tell someone how much enjoyment you get out of being together, in the biblical sense, with them, and the implication is that you wish to continue doing so, showing in another manner that you will be around for as long as you are able.

84. You love being fucked like a naughty little girl, don't you?

85. You love it when I stretch you open with my cock, don't you?

86. I love sucking your cock, and I'm going to lick you clean.

Telling your partner what you want to do, and being so explicit about the act can be done in the middle of the act itself, or beforehand as a look into what will happen next, causing all kinds of lovely mental images and increasing their desire and anticipation of what is to come exponentially.

87. I love how big your cock gets, how much this turns me on.

This offers another way to stroke a man's ego, and serves as not only validation, but boosts self-confidence enormously; the increased confidence level will make them more likely to do other things that they may have been on the fence about doing previously.

88. The sounds you make drive me crazy.

This phrase serves to encourage your partner to not only make more noise, but assures them that they are not making any weird or off-putting noises, easing any worry or apprehension they may have had about the sounds that were coming out of their mouths. No one wants to worry that they may sound like an injured kitten in the middle of sex.

89. I'm going to fuck you until you can't walk.

The inherent vulgarity provided by this statement can cause your partner to catch their breath, for all that it implies, and all the different scenarios that can be imagined off of these few simple words. Words or phrases that cause your partner's breath to catch should be noted, as those are the things that not only have caught them off guard, but are also things that they find particularly appealing.

90. I'm so fucking wet.

Another phrase that shows your partner how much you desire them specifically, which in turn gets them even hotter, and thus the cycle continues. You show them that they are the one who matters, and no one else, and that your desire is a direct result of their particular actions.

91. Let's see how many times I can make you come.

Another statement that can cause your partner's breath to hitch as they fantasize about you specifically and all the different things that you can, and will, do to and for them. This particular phrase can be especially effective when whispered softly into the ear, followed by trailing down their neck, lips barely, if at all, brushing against their skin.

92. Baby, don't stop. I love it when you do that.

Encouragement, encouragement, encouragement. If you want something to keep happening, if you want your partner to continue doing something, the key is to let them know how much you want it, how much you absolutely crave that touch, that motion, that action.

93. Oh god, oh my fucking god.

Sometimes coherent words just don't exist, and in that case, this old standby will always work to show that you're just this side of starting to lose complete and total coherency as a result of whatever it is they are doing.

94. That's right, ride my hand.

It's one thing to be teased, it's quite another to be told to continue to tease yourself, and the thrill that comes not only from being told to do so, but to use your partner's hand to do so dramatically increases the effect.

95. Do you want more? Beg me for it.

By asking a question and then telling them how to answer, you are showing that you are the one in control of the show; you are the one who calls all the shots, and if they want something to happen, they will have to submit, at least for now, to doing it your way. This is an incredible turn on for either partner.

96. Take it.

Telling your partner to take everything you've got as you increase the intensity of your action is a very powerful feeling, a very primal feeling, which serves to bring out the slightly animalistic side in humans and serves to intensify the sensations themselves as they respond back, asking, demanding, begging for everything you're willing to give.

97. Fuck me. Right now.

Another real ego booster, showing that no matter what, any further delay, even that of a second will be far too long, and you cannot wait, desire nothing more, than to fuck them then and there, regardless of where you are, or who may be around.

98. I want you to use me as your toy all night long.

Once more, this phrasing not only shows that you are giving up control to your partner, but also shows the level of trust that you have in your partner; that they will make it a mutually beneficial and mutually enjoyable experience, as opposed to leaving one party feeling like they're being used.

99. Fill me up with your big dick; fuck my tight cunt.

Not only does this particular turn of phrase serve as an ego boost for both of you, it also provides explicit descriptions that will serve to excite both partners, and enhance the overall experience.

100. You can have me any way you want me.

This is another phrase that can be used to give up control to your partner and show that you have the utmost trust in them, that they will not hurt you, or abuse you in any way, and that they will ensure that both of you have a very good time.

101. Spread your legs for me.

This command serves to show who will be the dominant party for this particular time, or through the course of the following specific actions, demanding that they open to you, not only physically, but mentally as well. It ensures that both partners are right there where the actions are taking place, as opposed to lost in their own heads.

102. Faster!

This shows that you are getting closer and closer to exploding, and the closer you get, the more friction you want, which will in turn cause them to pick up their pace due to increased arousal from hearing this one simple word come out of your mouth.

103. I want you to use that big dick of yours to make me scream.

Expressing the exact actions you want your partner to take, while at the same time providing specific cause and effect actions with the appropriate adjectives to again provide an ego boost serves to augment the already intense feelings that are present.

104. What a sweet, sexy ass; I'm going to put it to good use.

First the compliment is provided on a particular body part, serving to decrease any self-confidence issues that may be present, and then the declarative statement that the particular body part in question is about to be utilized in one or more of the many different ways that it can be utilized is a definite mood enhancer.

105. I'm going to fuck you whenever I want, wherever I want.

This possessive declarative statement causes things to tighten deep in the body, showing that your partner desires you, and they will have you when and where they want, regardless of the potential consequences that may result due to these actions, because their desire is just that great.

106. Bend over.

These two simple words cause a surge of anticipation, as the person to whom they are spoken does not know what will happen next. They may have been bad and need a spanking, or perhaps they are going to get fucked in one of several different ways, or perhaps they are simply being told to do so as a method of waiting, causing the tension and desire levels to continue to rise.

107. I love the sounds you make when I touch you here.

Once more, this offers up the assurances that the noises that your partner is making do not cause them to sound like a disgruntled guinea pig, and indicates that you have made note of a particularly erogenous zone on their body. It allows you to both soothe any potential worries away while bringing attention to the fact that you have noticed the particular area in question that causes them to squirm.

108. Fuck my brains out.

This explicit statement shows that your desire levels cannot get much higher and you are just aching for your partner. You can't take much more teasing, and you want them right then, right there, and right now, regardless of where you are or how many people may or not be around.

109. Make me.

This defiant little statement just begs for your partner to put you in your place, take control of the situation, and dominate you, bending your actions to his whim. It's just the right amount of saucy to not sound like a whiney little two year old, and just the right amount of defiant to make the taming especially fun.

110. Tell me how much you like my cock.

This works to get your partner to be more vocal, and serves as a way to combine the picture that the words paint with the visual that is taking place at that exact point in time, which serves to enhance the experience itself. It also serves to show your partner how much you are enjoying yourself, and provides a nice ego boost for you.

111. If you keep that up, I'm going to come.

This simple declaration tells your partner that not only are they doing something very, very right, but how close you are to coming all over (insert object here). They can then choose whether or not they want to continue and allow you to climax, or slow down to prolong the teasing and deliciously aching agony.

112. You like this, don't you?

A phrase like this one demands active engagement from your partner, demanding they tell you what their feelings are on a particular action. It makes sure that they are thinking about nothing other than what is going on right then and there with you, that they are fully cognizant of all that is going on around them, and provides an affirmation of what is being done oh so very right and what could use a little work.

113. I'm ready to go again.

This lets your partner know that it was not a one off thing, you still want them just as much as you did before, and you don't want to be separated, but rather would prefer to continue with everything that you both have got.

114. I can't get enough of you.

This tells your partner that no matter how long you have been together, or how many times you have been together, you still want them just as much as you did the first day, if not more than you did when you first met. It shows them in another way how truly awesome they really are in your book.

115. That was the best fuck I've ever had.

As mentioned before, comparative statements are always best to shy away from, but well, when something is true, it's true, and due to the insecurities of most people, this will probably serve to boost their confidence levels sky high.

116. You've been a very naughty girl. I'm going to wash your mouth out with my cum for being such a dirty girl.

This goes off of the dominant/submissive aspects of sex, and the "bad girl" persona, one who has been very naughty, needs to be punished, and provides a pleasant form of punishment that shows who is dominant, but gives both parties something very enjoyable to do in that context.

117. You've been a bad girl, and you deserve a spanking.

This too goes into the dominant submissive aspects that can be present in a particular relationship, and shows that one has power over the other, while providing just enough of a sting to bring about intense pleasure in both parties.

118. Get on your hands and knees, sweetheart...and wait like a good girl.

This shows dominance by the other partner, and heightens the arousal of both parties with the addition of the waiting aspect. The person who is forced to wait on their hands and knees does not know what will happen next, causing them to imagine all different sorts of fantasies, and the person who gave the instruction will savor the anticipation being felt by their partner, gleefully determining what their next course of action will be.

119. Don't you dare come until I say you can.

This form of command demands that your partner attempt to exert some form of control over their own bodies, and the attempt to do so, in spite of the sensations being felt by their own body is almost enough to push them over the edge through the direct result of the very thought process attempting to prevent that from occurring. While that kind of control can eventually be learned, it is not required in order for this phrasing to not only work, but to add some spice into your love life.

120. I'm going to make you come until you can't breathe.

As the turn of phrase states, "There should be a word for a threat that is also a promise, for that is what I want to do to you." If there was such a word, it would apply to this particular phrasing, guaranteeing their breath to catch, their heart to race, and their imaginations to go wild, attempting to determine all the different ways that this particular action will occur.

During Orgasm

121. Come in my mouth. I promise not to spill a drop.

This conveys further images of the naughty, but "good" girl, who doesn't waste a thing, showing how much she likes the particular act, that she enjoys how you taste, and desires to have the power rush that comes from making someone else come as a result of oral sex.

122. Come really hard for me.

123. Come on that cock.

This command is enough to send just about anyone straight over the edge. It has the flavor of one person being dominant over the other, by virtue of commanding the other person to a particular action, but the carnality of it is what serves to push it straight over the edge. This is also something that is typically said right before the other party is about to come, and with the right inflection and commanding tone in the voice it can serve to have you and your partner coming at the exact same time and increasing the closeness felt, and the depth of the intensity that is felt.

124. Keep coming hard for me.

125. Come on my tits.

This provides a visual image to go along with the description, coming unbidden to mind immediately upon utterance, and gives your partner a feeling of power by marking you, even though you were the one to tell them what to do.

126. I want you to come all over me.

127. You want to come for me, don't you?

128. You're going to come so hard you're going to wet the bed.

129. Where do you want me to come?

This not only asks permission, requests a command, but also provides many different visuals in addition to letting your partner know that you are close to reaching that pinnacle. It also shows a potential shift back to the normal relationship dynamics, from the different dynamics present during the act itself.

130. Come inside of me.

Regardless of the type of protection used or not used, this has the connotations attached to it that show that you are willing to remain with that person, no matter what, come what may, and you want both of you to experience that utmost completeness that is felt when one person comes while still inside of another.

131. Come for me.

This three word command is usually enough to send just about anyone straight over the edge, and is usually used when the other partner is close to coming so that both may do so at the same time. It shows which partner is the dominant party, and serves to provide a heightened anticipation and excitement for both parties.

Final Thoughts

I hope that these different examples have provided more than an ample amount of ways to get you started, not just with thinking about the topic, but imagining how this could best be mixed in to your lives. These are by no means the only different things that you can say, nor are they perhaps the phrasing that you personally would use, or even the spelling you would normally use, but they should have served as a means and a way to not only get you started thinking about the different things that you want to say, or the different things you want to hear. You may even show this particular article to your partner and use it as a means of bringing up the subject to them! By looking at the reasons behind why certain things work, you should be able to go through and figure out more about the type of person you are in bed, and what you like, which will not only serve to increase your pleasure, but increase your partner's pleasure as well.

Each and every person is going to have a different form of dirty talk. Some people prefer the tamer variations on different things that they can say, while other prefer the vulgar; the more vulgar the better; the more coarse the better. Regardless of whether you prefer tame, or if it's the hardcore dirty talk that really rings your bell, either version, either way, is completely okay and perfectly natural. There is no good or bad way to talk dirty to your partner. The important thing is that it is natural for you to say, that you do not get embarrassed as a result of the things that you say, and that you work to incorporate the phrases and methods that you want to use into your life in the way that works best for you. Some people may not choose to take it to text messages or to emails, while others will keep it only in text and never utter a word out loud, but whatever the method used, whatever the medium used, and whatever the intensity used, it is all completely acceptable.

Sex is a taboo subject in our society; it is used to sell everything, but it is never discussed openly, and because of that, many different people are concerned with, or unsure of, how to get started bringing dirty talk into their sex lives. As long as you are comfortable with the level you use, the words you use, and enjoy how it makes you feel, then you are doing it right. What may flat out do it for one person may be completely cheesy and ridiculous to another, and that's okay too. Every different person has different kinks, quirks, and preferences in regards to their sexuality, and the sexuality of their partners, as long as you are all satisfied and have a happy and healthy sex life (and you remember not to send naughty or not safe for work emails to your partner's company email address) you should be more than set. We wish you the best of luck in spicing up your sex life and hope that this has been helpful and informative for you.

Other books by Elizabeth Cramer:

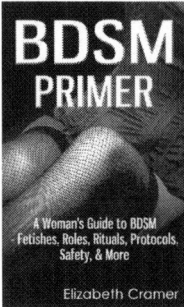

BDSM Primer - A Woman's Guide to BDSM - Fetishes, Roles, Rituals, Protocols, Safety, & More

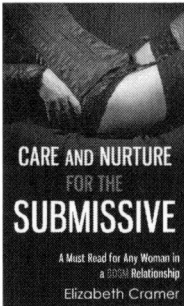

Care and Nurture for the Submissive - A Must Read for Any Woman in a BDSM Relationship

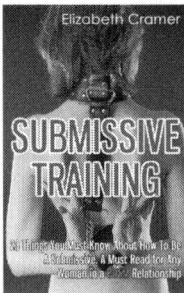

Submissive Training: 23 Things You Must Know About How To Be A Submissive. A Must Read For Any Woman In A BDSM Relationship

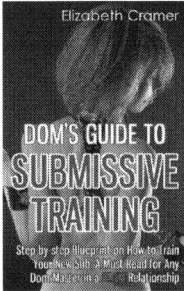

Dom's Guide To Submissive Training: Step-by-step Blueprint On How To Train Your New Sub. A Must Read For Any Dom/Master In A BDSM Relationship

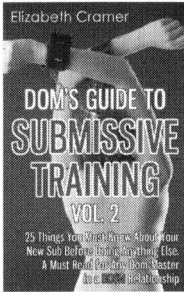

Dom's Guide To Submissive Training Vol. 2: 25 Things You Must Know About Your New Sub Before Doing Anything Else. A Must Read For Any Dom/Master In A BDSM Relationship

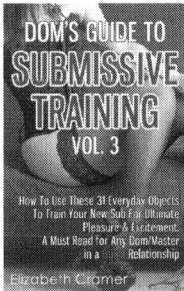

Dom's Guide To Submissive Training Vol. 3: How To Use These 31 Everyday Objects To Train Your New Sub For Ultimate Pleasure & Excitement. A Must Read For Any Dom/Master In A BDSM Relationship

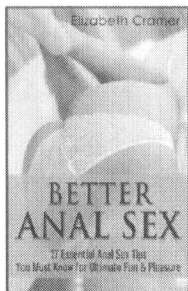

Better Anal Sex - 27 Essential Anal Sex Tips You Must Know for Ultimate Fun & Pleasure

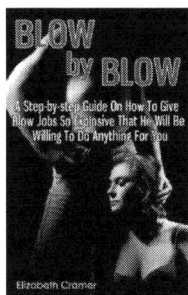

Blow By Blow - A Step-by-step Guide On How To Give Blow Jobs So Explosive That He Will Be Willing To Do Anything For You

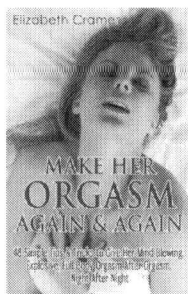

Make Her Orgasm Again and Again: 48 Simple Tips & Tricks to Give Her Mind-Blowing, Explosive, Full-Body Orgasm After Orgasm, Night After Night

17930714R00044

Printed in Great Britain
by Amazon